NO GALLBLADDER COOKBOOK FOR WOMEN

35 Quick and Easy Tasty Recipes for Your Healthy Living

MEY W SMITH

TABLE OF

Introduction

The No Gallbladder Cookbook for women is a valuable resource designed to address the unique dietary needs of individuals who have undergone gallbladder removal surgery. This cookbook aims to provide delicious and nutritious recipes that support digestion and overall well-being in the absence of the gallbladder.

Types of Gallbladder Issues in Women

Gallbladder issues affecting women often include gallstones, inflammation, or the need for gallbladder removal due to complications. Post-surgery, individuals may experience challenges in digesting certain foods, making dietary adjustments crucial for maintaining health.

Causes of Gallbladder Issues in Women

Several factors contribute to gallbladder problems in women. These may include a diet high in cholesterol and fat, obesity, rapid weight loss, or hormonal changes, particularly during pregnancy. Genetic predisposition and certain medical conditions can also increase the risk of gallbladder issues.

Symptoms of Gallbladder Issues in Women

Common symptoms of gallbladder problems in women include abdominal pain, especially in the upper right portion, nausea, vomiting, and digestive discomfort after consuming fatty or greasy foods. Women may also experience bloating, indigestion, and changes in bowel habits.

Preventive Measures for Gallbladder Issues in Women

1. -Healthy Diet:- Adopting a diet low in saturated fats and cholesterol can help prevent gallstone formation. The No Gallbladder Cookbook emphasizes recipes that are easy on the digestive system while providing essential nutrients.

2. -Regular Exercise:- Engaging in regular physical activity promotes overall health and can contribute to weight management, reducing the risk of gallbladder issues.

3. -Hydration:- Drinking an adequate amount of water supports digestion and helps in preventing the formation of gallstones.

4. -Moderate Weight Loss:- If weight loss is necessary, gradual and steady methods are recommended to avoid triggering gallstone formation.

5. -Balanced Hormones:- For women, maintaining hormonal balance, especially during pregnancy and menopause, can help prevent gallbladder problems associated with hormonal fluctuations.

6. -Consultation with Healthcare Provider:- Regular check-ups and consultation with a healthcare provider can help identify and address potential gallbladder issues early on.

the No Gallbladder Cookbook for women serves as a valuable guide in navigating dietary challenges post-gallbladder removal. By understanding the types, causes, symptoms, and adopting preventive measures, women can manage their health effectively and enjoy a fulfilling lifestyle. Always consult with a healthcare professional for personalized advice and recommendations based on individual health conditions.

Chapter 1

What to eat and not

The No Gallbladder Cookbook for women offers a thoughtful approach to meal planning, focusing on foods that support digestive health and minimize discomfort after gallbladder removal surgery. Understanding which foods to include and avoid becomes crucial in managing the unique challenges of living without a gallbladder.

Foods to Include

1. -Lean Proteins:- Opt for lean protein sources such as poultry, fish, and tofu. These proteins are easier to digest and place less strain on the digestive system.

2. -Fiber-Rich Foods:- Include plenty of fruits, vegetables, and whole grains in your diet. High-fiber foods aid digestion and help prevent constipation, a common concern after gallbladder removal.

3. -Healthy Fats:- Choose sources of healthy fats, such as avocados, nuts, seeds, and olive oil. These fats are easier on the digestive system compared to saturated fats found in fried and processed foods.

4. -Low-Fat Dairy:- Select low-fat or fat-free dairy products to reduce the intake of saturated fats. Incorporate options like skim milk, yogurt, and cheese in moderation.

5. -Small, Frequent Meals:- Instead of three large meals, consider consuming smaller, more frequent meals throughout the day. This approach helps manage digestion by avoiding overloading the digestive system.

6. -Hydrating Beverages:- Drink plenty of water to stay well-hydrated. Herbal teas and diluted fruit juices can also be included, but caffeinated and carbonated beverages should be consumed in moderation.

7. -Herbs and Spices:- Flavor meals with herbs and spices like ginger, turmeric, and mint. These not only enhance the taste but also offer potential digestive benefits.

-Foods to Avoid:-

1. -High-Fat Foods:- Limit or avoid high-fat foods, as the gallbladder is responsible for storing bile that aids in fat digestion. Without a gallbladder, the body may struggle to process large amounts of fat, leading to digestive discomfort. This includes fried foods, fatty meats, and rich desserts.

2. -Processed Foods:- Reduce intake of processed and packaged foods, as they often contain unhealthy fats,

preservatives, and additives that can be challenging for digestion.

3. -Spicy Foods:- Some individuals may find that spicy foods can trigger digestive issues, so it's advisable to moderate the consumption of spicy dishes.

4. -Caffeine and Carbonated Drinks:- Excessive caffeine intake and carbonated beverages can contribute to digestive discomfort and should be consumed in moderation.

5. -Highly Acidic Foods:- Citrus fruits and acidic foods may cause irritation for some individuals. Pay attention to how your body responds and adjust your intake accordingly.

6. -Large Meals:- Avoid consuming large meals, which can overwhelm the digestive system. Opt for smaller, more frequent meals to promote smoother digestion.

7. -Alcohol:- Limit alcohol consumption, as it can stress the liver and digestive system. If you choose to drink, do so in moderation and pay attention to how your body reacts.

In conclusion, the No Gallbladder Cookbook for women encourages a balanced and mindful approach to eating, emphasizing whole, nutrient-dense foods while avoiding those that may strain the digestive system. It's essential to listen to your body's signals and make adjustments based on individual responses. Consulting with a healthcare professional or a nutritionist can provide personalized guidance to ensure optimal digestive health after gallbladder removal.

Benefits

Following a diet based on the No Gallbladder Cookbook for women can offer several core benefits, providing a tailored approach to nutrition that supports overall health and well-being after gallbladder removal. Here are some key advantages:

1. -Digestive Comfort:- The cookbook emphasizes foods that are easier to digest, helping to prevent discomfort and digestive issues commonly experienced after gallbladder surgery. By selecting easily digestible options, individuals can reduce the risk of bloating, gas, and indigestion.

2. -Balanced Fat Intake:- Since the gallbladder is responsible for storing bile, which aids in fat digestion, managing fat intake becomes crucial after its removal. The cookbook guides women in choosing healthy fats and moderating overall fat consumption, promoting a balanced approach that minimizes the risk of fatty food-induced discomfort.

3. -Nutrient-Dense Choices:- The recipes in the cookbook focus on nutrient-dense ingredients, ensuring that

individuals receive essential vitamins and minerals necessary for overall health.

This approach helps prevent nutritional deficiencies that may arise due to changes in digestion post-gallbladder surgery.

4. -Stable Blood Sugar Levels:- The cookbook advocates for a balanced diet that includes complex carbohydrates, lean proteins, and healthy fats. This balanced approach can contribute to stable blood sugar levels, preventing spikes and crashes that may affect energy levels and overall well-being.

5. -Weight Management:- The emphasis on portion control and choosing nutrient-dense foods can aid in weight management. Maintaining a healthy weight is essential for overall health and can reduce the risk of complications associated with obesity, which may exacerbate gallbladder issues.

6. -Improved Bowel Regularity:- The inclusion of fiber-rich foods in the cookbook promotes bowel regularity, preventing constipation that may occur after gallbladder removal. Fiber helps in maintaining healthy digestion and supporting the overall function of the digestive tract.

7. -Hydration:- Proper hydration is crucial for digestion and overall health. The cookbook encourages the consumption of hydrating foods and beverages, helping individuals stay

well-hydrated, which is essential for various bodily functions.

8. -Reduced Risk of Gallstone Formation:- By focusing on a diet that minimizes the intake of high-fat and processed foods, the cookbook aims to reduce the risk of gallstone formation. This is particularly important for preventing complications in individuals who have undergone gallbladder removal surgery.

9. -Increased Energy Levels:- A well-balanced diet contributes to sustained energy levels throughout the day. By providing the body with the necessary nutrients, the cookbook supports overall vitality and helps individuals avoid energy slumps often associated with poor dietary choices.

10. -Psychological Well-being:- Following a diet tailored to the needs of individuals without a gallbladder can alleviate anxiety and stress related to digestive discomfort. Knowing which foods to include and avoid provides a sense of control over one's health, positively impacting psychological well-being.

The No Gallbladder Cookbook for women offers a holistic approach to nutrition, addressing not only the physical aspects of digestive health but also promoting overall well-being. By incorporating the core principles outlined in the cookbook, women can enjoy improved digestion, nutrient intake, and a better quality of life after gallbladder removal.

Shopping ingredients

1. -Lean Proteins:-
   - Skinless poultry (chicken or turkey)
   - Fish (salmon, trout, cod)
   - Tofu or tempeh for plant-based protein options

2. -Low-Fat Dairy:-
   - Skim milk or lactose-free milk
   - Low-fat yogurt
   - Reduced-fat cheese

3. -Whole Grains:-
   - Quinoa
   - Brown rice
   - Oats

4. -Healthy Fats:-
   - Avocados
   - Nuts (almonds, walnuts)
   - Seeds (flaxseeds, chia seeds)

5. -Fruits:-
   - Berries (blueberries, strawberries)

- Apples
- Bananas

6. -Vegetables:-
    - Leafy greens (spinach, kale)
    - Cruciferous vegetables (broccoli, cauliflower)
    - Bell peppers

7. -Herbs and Spices:-
    - Ginger
    - Turmeric
    - Mint
    - Basil

8. -Whole Foods for Fiber:-
    - Legumes (lentils, chickpeas)
    - Beans (black beans, kidney beans)

9. -Hydrating Beverages:-
    - Water
    - Herbal teas (peppermint, chamomile)

10. -Lean Cuts of Meat:-
    - Lean cuts of beef (sirloin, tenderloin)
    - Pork loin

11. -Non-Citrus Fruits:-
    - Papaya

- Melons (watermelon, cantaloupe)

12. -Non-Gassy Vegetables:-
   - Zucchini
   - Cucumbers
   - Carrots

13. -Whole Wheat Products:-
   - Whole wheat bread
   - Whole wheat pasta

14. -Low-Fat Salad Dressings:-
   - Olive oil-based dressings
   - Balsamic vinegar

15. -Low-Fat Soups:-
   - Vegetable-based soups
   - Broth-based soups with lean protein

16. -Eggs:-
   - Eggs provide a versatile and easily digestible protein source.

17. -Dried Herbs for Flavoring:-
   - Dried oregano
   - Dill
   - Rosemary

18. -Non-Acidic Tomatoes:-
   - Cherry tomatoes
   - Roma tomatoes

19. -Non-Citrus Juices:-
   - Apple juice
   - Pear juice

20. -Whole, Unprocessed Snacks:-
   - Hummus with vegetable sticks
   - Nut and seed mixes (in moderation)

These ingredients can form the basis for a variety of tasty and digestive-friendly recipes. When shopping, prioritize fresh, whole foods and read labels to avoid processed and high-fat items. Additionally, individual preferences and tolerances may vary, so it's advisable to pay attention to how your body reacts to different foods and adjust your choices accordingly. Consultation with a healthcare professional or nutritionist can provide personalized guidance based on specific dietary needs.

BREAKFAST

1. -Quinoa Breakfast Bowl

-Ingredients-
- 1 cup cooked quinoa
- 1/2 cup fresh berries (blueberries, strawberries)
- 1 tablespoon chopped nuts (almonds or walnuts)
- 1 tablespoon honey

-Preparation-
- Mix quinoa, berries, and nuts in a bowl.
- Drizzle honey on top.

-Nutritional Value-
- Protein: 8g, Fiber: 5g, Calories: 300
-Cooking Time-
- 15 minutes (assuming quinoa is pre-cooked).

2. Avocado Toast with Poached Egg

-Ingredients-
- 1 slice whole wheat bread
- 1/2 ripe avocado, mashed
- 1 poached egg
- Salt and pepper to taste

-Preparation-

- Toast the bread and spread mashed avocado.
- Top with a poached egg and season.

-Nutritional Value-
    - Protein: 12g, Fiber: 7g, Calories: 250
-Cooking Time-
    - 10 minutes.

3. Greek Yogurt Parfait

-Ingredients-
    - 1 cup low-fat Greek yogurt
    - 1/4 cup granola
    - 1/2 cup mixed berries
    - 1 tablespoon honey

-Preparation-
    - Layer yogurt, granola, and berries in a glass.
    - Drizzle honey on top.

-Nutritional Value-
    - Protein: 15g, Fiber: 4g, Calories: 280
-Cooking Time-
    - 5 minutes.

4. Veggie Omelette

-Ingredients-
    - 2 eggs

- 1/4 cup diced bell peppers
- 1/4 cup diced tomatoes
- 1/4 cup spinach
- Salt and pepper to taste

-Preparation-
- Whisk eggs and pour into a hot, non-stick pan.
- Add veggies, cook until set, and fold.

-Nutritional Value-
- Protein: 14g, Fiber: 3g, Calories: 220
-Cooking Time-
- 10 minutes.

5. Chia Seed Pudding

-Ingredients-
- 2 tablespoons chia seeds
- 1 cup almond milk
- 1/2 teaspoon vanilla extract
- 1 tablespoon maple syrup

-Preparation-
- Mix chia seeds, almond milk, vanilla, and maple syrup.
- Refrigerate overnight.

-Nutritional Value-
- Protein: 6g, Fiber: 10g, Calories: 180

-Cooking Time-
- Overnight refrigeration.

6. Banana Almond Smoothie

-Ingredients-
- 1 ripe banana
- 1 cup almond milk
- 1 tablespoon almond butter
- Ice cubes (optional)

-Preparation-
- Blend banana, almond milk, and almond butter until smooth.
- Add ice if desired.

-Nutritional Value-
- Protein: 7g, Fiber: 3g, Calories: 220
-Cooking Time-
- 5 minutes.

7. Cottage Cheese with Pineapple

-Ingredients-
- 1/2 cup low-fat cottage cheese
- 1/2 cup fresh pineapple chunks
- 1 tablespoon shredded coconut

-Preparation-
- Combine cottage cheese, pineapple, and coconut.

-Nutritional Value-
    - Protein: 14g, Fiber: 2g, Calories: 180
-Cooking Time-
    - 5 minutes.

8. Spinach and Feta Breakfast Wrap

-Ingredients-
    - 1 whole wheat tortilla
    - 2 eggs, scrambled
    - Handful of fresh spinach
    - 2 tablespoons crumbled feta cheese

-Preparation-
    - Fill tortilla with scrambled eggs, spinach, and feta.

-Nutritional Value-
    - Protein: 16g, Fiber: 4g, Calories: 290
-Cooking Time-
    - 10 minutes.

9. Sweet Potato Hash

-Ingredients-
    - 1 medium sweet potato, diced
    - 1/2 cup diced bell peppers
    - 1/4 cup diced onions
    - 1 tablespoon olive oil

-Preparation-
    - Sauté sweet potato, peppers, and onions in olive oil until tender.
-Nutritional Value-
    - Protein: 3g, Fiber: 4g, Calories: 180
-Cooking Time-
    - 15 minutes.

10. Blueberry Protein Pancakes

-Ingredients-
    - 1/2 cup oats (blended into flour)
    - 1/2 cup low-fat cottage cheese
    - 2 eggs
    - 1/2 cup blueberries

-Preparation-
    - Mix oat flour, cottage cheese, eggs, and fold in blueberries.
    - Cook as regular pancakes on a griddle.

-Nutritional Value-
    - Protein: 15g, Fiber: 3g, Calories: 280
-Cooking Time-
    - 15 minutes.

These recipes offer a variety of nutritious options to start the day, considering the specific dietary needs of women without a gallbladder. Adjust portions based on individual preferences and consult with a healthcare professional for personalized guidance.

LUNCH

1. Grilled Chicken Salad

-Ingredients-
- 4 oz grilled chicken breast, sliced
- 2 cups mixed salad greens
- 1/2 cup cherry tomatoes, halved
- 1/4 cup cucumber, sliced
- 2 tablespoons balsamic vinaigrette

-Preparation-
- Arrange salad greens, top with chicken, tomatoes, and cucumber.
- Drizzle with balsamic vinaigrette.

-Nutritional Value-
- Protein: 25g, Fiber: 4g, Calories: 300
-Cooking Time-
- 15 minutes (grilling).

2. Quinoa and Vegetable Stir-Fry

-Ingredients-
- 1 cup cooked quinoa
- 1 cup mixed stir-fry vegetables (broccoli, bell peppers, snap peas)
- 2 tablespoons low-sodium soy sauce

- 1 tablespoon sesame oil
-Preparation-
    - Stir-fry vegetables, add cooked quinoa, soy sauce, and sesame oil.

-Nutritional Value-
    - Protein: 10g, Fiber: 5g, Calories: 250
-Cooking Time-
    - 15 minutes.

3. Lentil and Vegetable Soup

-Ingredients-
    - 1/2 cup dry lentils
    - 2 cups mixed vegetables (carrots, celery, zucchini)
    - 1/2 cup diced tomatoes
    - 4 cups vegetable broth

-Preparation-
    - Cook lentils and vegetables in broth until tender.
-Nutritional Value-
    - Protein: 12g, Fiber: 8g, Calories: 220
-Cooking Time-
    - 30 minutes.

4. Turkey Lettuce Wraps

-Ingredients-
    - 4 oz ground turkey

- 1/2 cup black beans, drained and rinsed
- 1/4 cup diced tomatoes
- Lettuce leaves for wrapping

-Preparation-
- Cook ground turkey, mix with black beans and tomatoes.
- Spoon into lettuce leaves.

-Nutritional Value-
- Protein: 20g, Fiber: 6g, Calories: 280
-Cooking Time-
- 15 minutes.

5. Quinoa and Chickpea Salad

-Ingredients-
- 1 cup cooked quinoa
- 1/2 cup chickpeas, drained and rinsed
- 1/2 cup cucumber, diced
- 1/4 cup feta cheese, crumbled
- 2 tablespoons olive oil

-Preparation-
- Combine quinoa, chickpeas, cucumber, and feta.
- Drizzle with olive oil.

-Nutritional Value-

- Protein: 12g, Fiber: 6g, Calories: 260
-Cooking Time-
    - 15 minutes.

6. Baked Salmon with Lemon-Dill Sauce

-Ingredients-
    - 6 oz salmon fillet
    - 1 tablespoon fresh dill, chopped
    - 1 tablespoon lemon juice
    - Salt and pepper to taste

-Preparation-
    - Season salmon with dill, lemon juice, salt, and pepper.
    - Bake until cooked through.

-Nutritional Value-
    - Protein: 28g, Fiber: 1g, Calories: 300
-Cooking Time-
    - 20 minutes (baking).

7. Veggie and Hummus Wrap

-Ingredients-
    - 1 whole wheat tortilla
    - 2 tablespoons hummus
    - 1/2 cup mixed vegetables (bell peppers, carrots, cucumbers)

-Preparation-

- Spread hummus on the tortilla, top with vegetables.
- Roll into a wrap.

-Nutritional Value-
- Protein: 8g, Fiber: 5g, Calories: 220

-Cooking Time-
- 5 minutes.

8. Shrimp and Quinoa Bowl

-Ingredients-
- 4 oz shrimp, peeled and deveined
- 1 cup cooked quinoa
- 1/2 cup cherry tomatoes, halved
- 1/4 cup avocado, diced

-Preparation-
- Sauté shrimp until cooked, serve over quinoa.
- Top with tomatoes and avocado.

-Nutritional Value-
- Protein: 20g, Fiber: 5g, Calories: 280

-Cooking Time-
- 15 minutes.

9. Caprese Salad with Chicken

-Ingredients-
- 4 oz grilled chicken breast, sliced
- 1 cup cherry tomatoes, halved

- 1/2 cup fresh mozzarella, diced
- Fresh basil leaves
- Balsamic glaze for drizzling

-Preparation-
    - Arrange chicken, tomatoes, and mozzarella.
    - Garnish with basil and drizzle with balsamic glaze.

-Nutritional Value-
    - Protein: 24g, Fiber: 3g, Calories: 320
-Cooking Time-
    - 15 minutes (grilling).

10. Turkey and Vegetable Skewers

-Ingredients-
    - 4 oz turkey breast, cut into chunks
    - Bell peppers, cherry tomatoes, and zucchini chunks
    - Olive oil, garlic, and herbs for marinating

-Preparation-
    - Marinate turkey and vegetables in olive oil, garlic, and
herbs.
    - Skewer and grill until cooked through.

-Nutritional Value-
    - Protein: 22g, Fiber: 4g, Calories: 290

-Cooking Time-
- 20 minutes (grilling).

These recipes provide a diverse range of options for a nutritious and gallbladder-friendly lunch. Adjust portions based on individual preferences and consult with a healthcare professional for personalized guidance.

DINNER

1. Grilled Lemon Herb Chicken

-Ingredients-
- 6 oz chicken breast
- 1 tablespoon olive oil
- 1 teaspoon lemon zest
- Fresh herbs (rosemary, thyme)

-Preparation-
- Marinate chicken in olive oil, lemon zest, and herbs.
- Grill until cooked through.

-Nutritional Value-
- Protein: 30g, Fiber: 1g, Calories: 350
-Cooking Time-
- 15 minutes (grilling).

2. Baked Cod with Tomato Salsa

-Ingredients-

- 6 oz cod fillet
- 1 cup cherry tomatoes, diced
- 1/4 cup red onion, finely chopped
- 1 tablespoon fresh cilantro, chopped

-Preparation-
- Place cod in a baking dish, top with tomato salsa.
- Bake until fish is flaky.
-Nutritional Value-
- Protein: 28g, Fiber: 2g, Calories: 280
-Cooking Time-
- 20 minutes (baking).

3. Quinoa Stuffed Bell Peppers

-Ingredients-
- 1 cup cooked quinoa
- 2 bell peppers, halved
- 1/2 cup black beans, drained and rinsed
- 1/4 cup corn kernels

-Preparation-
- Mix quinoa, black beans, and corn.
- Stuff bell peppers and bake until peppers are tender.

-Nutritional Value-
- Protein: 12g, Fiber: 6g, Calories: 250
-Cooking Time-

- 25 minutes (baking).

4. Eggplant and Chickpea Curry

-Ingredients-
- 1 large eggplant, diced
- 1 can chickpeas, drained
- 1 onion, finely chopped
- 2 tomatoes, diced

-Preparation-
- Sauté onion, add eggplant, chickpeas, and tomatoes.
- Simmer until vegetables are tender.

-Nutritional Value-
- Protein: 10g, Fiber: 8g, Calories: 220
-Cooking Time-
- 30 minutes.

5. Shrimp and Vegetable Stir-Fry

-Ingredients-
- 6 oz shrimp, peeled and deveined
- 2 cups mixed stir-fry vegetables (broccoli, snap peas, carrots)
- 1 tablespoon low-sodium soy sauce

-Preparation-

- Stir-fry shrimp and vegetables in soy sauce until cooked.

-Nutritional Value-
    - Protein: 20g, Fiber: 4g, Calories: 280
-Cooking Time-
    - 15 minutes.

6. Roasted Sweet Potato and Chickpea Bowl

-Ingredients-
    - 1 medium sweet potato, cubed
    - 1 can chickpeas, drained
    - 1 tablespoon olive oil
    - 1/2 teaspoon cumin

-Preparation-
    - Toss sweet potato and chickpeas in olive oil and cumin.
    - Roast until golden and tender.

-Nutritional Value-
    - Protein: 10g, Fiber: 6g, Calories: 250
-Cooking Time-
    - 30 minutes (roasting).

7. Turkey and Vegetable Skillet

-Ingredients-
- 8 oz ground turkey
- 1 cup mixed vegetables (bell peppers, zucchini, carrots)
- 1/2 cup tomato sauce
- Italian herbs and garlic for seasoning

-Preparation-
- Cook ground turkey, add vegetables, tomato sauce, and season.

-Nutritional Value-
- Protein: 24g, Fiber: 5g, Calories: 320

-Cooking Time-
- 20 minutes.

8. Cauliflower Fried Rice

-Ingredients-
- 2 cups cauliflower rice
- 1/2 cup peas and carrots, mixed
- 2 eggs, scrambled
- 1 tablespoon low-sodium soy sauce

-Preparation-
- Sauté cauliflower rice, add mixed veggies and eggs.
- Stir in soy sauce and cook until heated through.

-Nutritional Value-

- Protein: 12g, Fiber: 5g, Calories: 230
-Cooking Time-
    - 15 minutes.

9. Chicken and Spinach Stuffed Portobello Mushrooms

-Ingredients-
    - 2 large portobello mushrooms, stems removed
    - 6 oz cooked chicken breast, shredded
    - 1 cup fresh spinach, chopped
    - 1/4 cup feta cheese, crumbled

-Preparation-
    - Combine shredded chicken, spinach, and feta.
    - Stuff into mushrooms and bake until mushrooms are tender.

-Nutritional Value-
    - Protein: 26g, Fiber: 3g, Calories: 320
-Cooking Time-
    - 20 minutes (baking).

10. Lentil and Vegetable Curry

-Ingredients-
    - 1 cup dry lentils
    - 2 cups mixed vegetables (cauliflower, carrots, peas)

- 1 onion, finely chopped
- 1 can coconut milk

-Preparation-
- Cook lentils, sauté vegetables and onion, add coconut milk.
- Simmer until vegetables are tender.

-Nutritional Value-
- Protein: 14g, Fiber: 10g, Calories: 280
-Cooking Time-
- 30 minutes.

These dinner recipes provide a variety of flavorful and nutritious options tailored for women without a gallbladder. Adjust portions based on individual preferences and consult with a healthcare professional for personalized guidance.

SNACK

1. Greek Yogurt and Berry Parfait-

-Ingredients-
- 1 cup low-fat Greek yogurt
- 1/2 cup mixed berries (blueberries, strawberries)
- 2 tablespoons granola

-Preparation-
- Layer Greek yogurt, berries, and granola in a glass.

-Nutritional Value-
- Protein: 15g, Fiber: 4g, Calories: 220
-Preparation Time-
- 5 minutes.

2. Almond Butter Apple Slices

-Ingredients-
- 1 medium apple, sliced
- 2 tablespoons almond butter
- Cinnamon for sprinkling

-Preparation-
- Spread almond butter on apple slices and sprinkle with cinnamon.
-Nutritional Value-
- Protein: 4g, Fiber: 6g, Calories: 200

-Preparation Time-
- 3 minutes.

3. Veggie and Hummus Snack Plate

-Ingredients-
- 1/2 cup baby carrots
- 1/2 cucumber, sliced
- 1/2 bell pepper, sliced
- 3 tablespoons hummus

-Preparation-
- Arrange veggies on a plate with a side of hummus for dipping.

-Nutritional Value-
- Protein: 6g, Fiber: 5g, Calories: 150
-Preparation Time-
- 5 minutes.

4. Cottage Cheese with Pineapple and Walnuts

-Ingredients-
- 1/2 cup low-fat cottage cheese
- 1/2 cup fresh pineapple chunks
- 1 tablespoon chopped walnuts

-Preparation-
    - Combine cottage cheese, pineapple, and walnuts in a bowl.

-Nutritional Value-
    - Protein: 15g, Fiber: 2g, Calories: 220
-Preparation Time-
    - 3 minutes.

5. Avocado and Tomato Salsa Rice Cakes

-Ingredients-
    - 2 rice cakes
    - 1/2 avocado, mashed
    - 1/2 cup cherry tomatoes, diced
    - 1 tablespoon fresh cilantro, chopped

-Preparation-
    - Spread mashed avocado on rice cakes, top with tomato salsa.

-Nutritional Value-
    - Protein: 4g, Fiber: 3g, Calories: 180
-Preparation Time-
    - 5 minutes.

These snack recipes provide satisfying and gallbladder-friendly options for women. Adjust portions based on individual preferences and consult with a healthcare professional for personalized guidance.

Conclusion

The No Gallbladder Cookbook for women offers a tailored and thoughtful approach to nutrition, providing a wealth of recipes designed to support digestive health after gallbladder removal. By emphasizing easily digestible proteins, nutrient-dense options, and mindful choices, this cookbook addresses the unique dietary needs of women without a gallbladder. The recipes not only focus on preventing discomfort and digestive issues but also contribute to overall well-being.

The variety of breakfast, lunch, dinner, and snack options showcases the versatility and deliciousness that can be achieved within the confines of a gallbladder-friendly diet. From quinoa breakfast bowls to grilled lemon herb chicken, each recipe considers nutritional value, portion control, and the importance of incorporating a diverse range of ingredients to maintain a balanced diet.

Adopting and adapting to this specialized diet is not merely about managing the absence of a gallbladder; it's a journey toward nurturing your body with nourishing foods. By making these recipes a part of your routine, you are actively choosing a path that promotes digestive comfort, stable energy levels, and overall vitality. Moreover, this cookbook is not just a guide; it's an invitation to explore the world of flavors, textures, and nutrients that contribute to your well-being.

In embracing the No Gallbladder Cookbook, you are taking a step towards a healthier, more harmonious relationship with your body. It's an empowering decision that goes beyond the kitchen; it's a commitment to self-care and resilience. Remember, your health journey is unique, and this cookbook is a companion, offering support and encouragement as you navigate the path to a vibrant and fulfilling life post-gallbladder removal. With every meal, you are investing in your health and embracing the power of nourishment. Let the No Gallbladder Cookbook be your guide to a delicious and digestive-friendly lifestyle. Your body deserves the best – embrace this culinary adventure with enthusiasm and a sense of empowerment!

www.ingramcontent.com/pod-product-compliance
Lightning Source LLC
Chambersburg PA
CBHW070742260726
48660CB00007B/2938